Tara-Jayne has always known that her calling in life is to write books. While attending Kingston University, she studied creative writing and began learning more about her craft. Starting with script-writing and later blogging, Tara-Jayne has now written her first book focused on helping others reach their full potentials.

As a young black woman living in London, Tara-Jayne understands the day-to-day struggles of rejection and how detrimental this can be on your mindset. Armed with her religious beliefs and seeing positivity in every situation, this has allowed her to move forward and overcome personal battles such as grief and depression.

This book is dedicated to Beatrice Manufor, who raised me to always see the world positively. She left me with a mindset that focuses on inspiring others, and I hope this book will help those in constant battle with their own minds. I also want to thank all the practitioners who have produced amazing studies to assist us with transforming our mindset. Lastly, to all my readers, remember you can win in life because you hold all the control! It is after all YOUR mind!

Tara-Jayne Manufor

OK. NOW IT'S TIME TO GET YOUR MIND RIGHT!

30 AFFIRMATIONS TO STRENGTHEN YOUR MIND IN 30 DAYS

AUSTIN MACAULEY PUBLISHERS™

LONDON • CAMBRIDGE • NEW YORK • SHARJAH

A CIP catalogue record for this title is available from the British Library.

ISBN 9781528978491 (Paperback)
ISBN 9781528978514 (ePub e-book)

www.austinmacauley.com

First Published (2019)
Austin Macauley Publishers Ltd
25 Canada Square
Canary Wharf
London
E14 5LQ

Watch your thoughts, for they become words.
Watch your words, for they become actions.
Watch your actions, for they become habits.
Watch your habits, for they become character.
Watch your character, for it becomes your destiny.
— Lao Tzu

Introduction

This book has been written to support all of those experiencing difficulty with positive thinking. It will help change their mindset in thirty days with the help of daily affirmations.

My aim was to write a powerful and concise body of work that will inspire and bring strength to those in need. On life's journey, we need support and assistance from people who have been where we are and can share their winning strategies when dealing with life's hardships.

Have you ever felt like you are supposed to do more with your life but just settle in complacency?

You reject your own dreams and ambitions because your mind isn't strong enough to work towards a better life. We always moan that life is hard and grow miserable due to our constant daily challenges. Trust me, I am the biggest advocate for this! I quit, then start again, then quit and procrastinate and eventually lose all interest. This was until I realised the battle started in my mind and once I changed my outlook, everything else changed.

What we fail to understand is that life should be a battle! It is through trials and tribulations that we shape our character and become better, stronger people. We need to use these battles as learning curves to help prepare us for the next fight we will face.

This also relates to our success! Everyone wants to be successful but in reality, success doesn't usually happen overnight or with your first attempt at reaching your goal. You have to train your mind to revel in perseverance and use this determination as a motivation tool when aiming to reach a goal.

The path leading to success is not and should not be straightforward! We only really appreciate something we work hard towards and the same applies to achieving goals. The challenges we do not overcome when we give up, are the hurdles we need to face that assist in reaching our goal destination. You could be so close to reaching your goal but due to a negative thought process you give up and do not fulfil your full potential.

I like to believe we have to go through various battles to get us ready for the life that we are destined to have. There are many people who have not fulfilled their destinies due to losing their first major battle – conquering a losing mindset. When you believe within yourself that you have a winning life and your mind is made up to work towards reaching your goal, your outlook will be set to only see the best in every situation.

You see life through the eyes of a winner. For example, if you are in an accident, you may have lost your car but at least you did not lose your life. Use that incident as motivation to do something impactful with your life. You did not die which means you still have time to make a difference. You are here for a reason!

In order to grow, we need to make changes and change is never comfortable but it's definitely necessary. Change your mindset and you change your life.

"I will even make a way in the wilderness, and rivers in the desert," Isaiah 43:19.

God never gives you a burden you are not equipped to carry. Remember this the next time a challenge comes your way and your first thought is that of defeat.

Part One

Unlearning Fear – Power
of the Situation

Self-doubt starts in the mind but stems from a fear factor embedded in our hearts. The judgement of fear is an emotion we are all born with and its main purpose is to enable survival. Fear is a natural instinct but what we fear can be adjusted and negative behaviours unlearned. Learned, crippling, non-functional fear breeds negative thoughts and stops people from reaching their goals.

The brain plays an integral part when processing fear. Your brain will react with either a 'flight' or 'fight' response and this will determine how you deal with a fear. For example, you have never really been a fan of spiders and as you walk home and get to your front door, to your surprise you notice hanging above the frame a large spider.

Instantly, your sensory systems send signals to your brain that this is something to fear but where did this fear originate? How do you know you are actually afraid of spiders? Fear needs to come from somewhere and is usually something we inherit as children. This arachnophobia was initially implanted by your mother who would scream every time she saw a spider.

Caught in this pressing situation, your body begins to react to what your mind is telling it, and your adrenaline increases as your brain messages your heart rate requesting an increase, as well as instructing your sweat glands, to produce ample amounts. The reasoning response that is led from the higher cortical centre of the brain, then steps in and reminds you poisonous spiders do not live in this Country. Dependent on if you are swayed by your feelings, or logical reasoning will result in your actions. Will you brace the courage and step into your house, or will you call someone to come and save the day.

When we enter the world, we are born with two innate fears: The fear of falling and the fear of loud sounds. As infants we learn from the experiences influenced by our environment and cultures. Children learn what they fear based off the reactions and biases of their parents. If at a young age you are told that all dogs bite, you will automatically have a fear of dogs. You are unaware that trained dogs can be beautiful, loving companions, as you have only been fed the negative so only see the bad.

The same goes for if you touch something that is hot and get burnt. The pain that we associate with touching a pot on the stove sticks with us and we ensure we do not make the same mistake.

However, with age and growth we now know that if we are going to touch hot items, we have materials that aid us in completing our task. We can use oven gloves or a cloth once the flames are out to comply with fire safety. Either way, we have learnt to manoeuvre in a way where we can use our fear as an advancement rather than a limitation.

This happens when we understand how to unlearn fear. Unlearning fear is the difference between knowing what actually a threat to your life is, and what is an assumption you have made based on a negative experience. It's carefully readdressing all associations you have placed on something you are fearful.

Okay. So, how do we unlearn fear? The answer is programming. Brain stimulations bring past experiences to the forefront when we are faced with a situation. Situations motivate emotional reactions and the learned behaviours manifest and your mindset takes control. Dependent on whether you think positively or negatively, it will change the overall outcome of the situation.

I will revisit the power of a situation and the impact this has on your mindset, but first, let's delve further into our fear complexities and how to alter our fear memory.

Let's use the fear of dogs as an example. The learned fear needs to be replaced with a different experience associated with that fear in order to contradict what the brain expects from that fear. You need to install a new competitive memory. For instance, if you are given time alone with a puppy in a controlled environment, you will establish new memories that will modify your original fear memory. It is rare that this will happen on the first occasion but if you try this at least three times, you will begin to see your attitude change towards the learned fear.

Always remember, in order to readjust your learned fear association, you have to neutralise negative emotional meanings with positive experiences. The emotional part of our brains needs to experience a new association for your psyche to retrieve a lasting update.

As life is so uncertain, an uncontrolled situation will really test out this notion. Let us use a different type of phobia alongside the power of a situation for our next example.

Many known scenarios in life, related to a fear, don't always hold relevance to fears caused by personal insecurities. A personal insecurity can aid to anxiety which will preoccupy our minds with vague possibilities, in relation to a certain aspect of our lives or an uncomfortable situation.

Anxiety is one of the most dangerous affects caused by mismanaged fear. Anxiety equates to a fear of fear and is not something created to protect us from danger but rather from the advancement of life. Finding the root cause of the insecurity that causes the anxious phenomenon is extremely difficult but with support and in-depth self-analysation, it will prove beneficial and educational to assist with self-development and progression.

In the next example, we look at the fear of heartbreak and how your insecurities and mindset work in cohesion to determine your reactions and outlook in a situation. For many of us, matters of the heart are the hardest areas for us to let go of – past hurts. You could be stung in a business deal but continue to do business with other firms but once you feel heartbreak, opening up again is a struggle for some as we simply cannot forget the pain associated. Counter-productivity sets in and we build walls that serve as coping mechanisms. We assume that these walls are in place to protect us from future pain, but instead they act as barriers and leave us emotionally damaged and unavailable to those who have good intentions for our hearts. Finding a good balance is never easy as willingly walking down the road of vulnerability once you've been hurt is never an easy path to take.

The easiest technique to adopt in assisting this issue is to stop legislating rules on people. In life, we are determined to find a different outcome to a situation based on our behaviour. Our behaviours are influenced by our thought process and the relatable value we hold to a belief. This can be a belief about a person or a point of view about life and how it should be lived. The next example looks deeper at personal insecurities and how they can make or break a situation.

Sarah, a divorcee was previously involved in a marriage filled with infidelities. She was married to her ex-husband Michael for 10 years and it was revealed that he cheated multiple times. Sarah has now started dating Mark. Mark is hard working and spends a lot of time in the office. Their relationship has become very serious and Sarah has keys to Mark's house. On a whim, she decides to surprise him.

Sarah arrives to the house before Mark is back from work. She cooks dinner and patiently waits for him to return home. A car pulls up and Mark gets out. Sarah rushes to the window excited to see and surprise her man. As the car drives off, Sarah sees a woman behind the wheel.

Immediately, past experiences, vivid pictures and emotions flood Sarah's mind. She remembers all the pain she felt from her marriage and anger begins to build. Unexpectedly, we are thrown into a situation where two mindsets coincide with each other, both with a different outcome.

Negative Mindset Outcome

Sarah rushes over and opens the door. Mark smiles, surprised to see her. "Hi babe," he leans in to kiss her. Sarah pulls away.

"Hi babe!" she screeches engrossed with anger. "Hi babe!" she repeats and starts frantically pacing back and forth. "Mark honestly, do I look like I'm stupid and ready to have my heartbroken again!"

Mark looks on confused. He walks into the house. "What do you mean? I have no idea what you are talking about."

Sarah interrupts "Why are you lying? Why can't you just be honest? You're cheating on me! I saw the woman. I don't know why I thought you would be different." Mark walks towards the kitchen and sees two dinner plates neatly placed on the table.

"Oh. Now I know what this is about, Rebecca dropped me home, she's my…"

Sarah, clearly upset, continues muttering and grabs her coat. "Rebecca. OK. Well at least you were honest. This is all too much Mark, I can't go through lies and deceit again. I'm just done. I need to protect myself and clearly you're all the same," Sarah rushes out of the house. Mark stands in disbelief over the entire scenario. *What just happened?*

In the above example, Sarah allowed her learned behaviours inherited from her past to win. She did not take the time to reflect over the situation and ascertain concrete facts. She did not put the events into perspective and allowed her negative mindset to take control. This is the perfect route to disaster.

We can all remember a time where we have acted prematurely like Sarah. How did that end? On most occasions, negatively. In testing situations, overthinking with no factual evidence is the fastest way your mind works against you. Instead of automatically thinking that bad will happen, trust that only goodness is attracted to your life and you will deal with issues differently. As mentioned at the start of this chapter, you need to ensure your associations relating to a negative experience have transitioned into positive by creating new memories to replace the old. This will allow you to have a different leading perspective.

Personally, I have struggled with this and over the years have learnt that time is a healer for all wounds but the ultimate test is putting the theory into practice. We can read into all kinds of therapies and self-help books advising how to change our lives but unless we actually re-enact what we have read, what is the point? Unfortunately, until we understand and take responsibility for the damage our negative behaviours has on others, we will continue destroying any good that crosses our turbulent path. This tends to mostly happen when we have not transitioned from a past experience and are still in a dark, empty place within ourselves. There are many times where this can go unnoticed but how you react to situations can be a clear indicator. When we expect another person to fix us and fill in the empty voids caused by a painful past, a further danger occurs and does not assist with our healing process. This type of behaviour is counterproductive to our self-development and often leads to us unintentionally hurting an innocent person, who has no idea of the true extent of the fear that has led us to act inconsiderately.

However it doesn't have to end with us overreacting and our actions hurting people we care about. Let's look at what happens when our minds are disciplined and swayed more towards a positive thought process.

Positive Mindset Outcome

Sarah sits down. She takes a second to actively reason with her thoughts, "*Mark is not Michael. He hasn't done anything that would suspect me that he has been unfaithful. Why would he give me a key to his house if he wasn't serious? Let me just stay calm and hear him out.*" Mark walks in. He's surprised to see Sarah, "Hi babe."

Sarah smiles, "Hey. I thought I'd surprise you."

Mark walks towards Sarah "Well, it's a pleasant surprise," he kisses her. "Babe, I'm so happy to see you! Today has been so stressful! I didn't even want to take the train. Luckily, Rebecca from work was going to watch her daughter's school play and dropped me off. You know St Saviours at the end of the road, her children go there."

Sarah smiles to herself proud with how she dealt with her initial thoughts. "Yes I know it," Sarah relaxes.

So, the same situation results a different outcome due to a different mindset. Everyone has the capabilities of making a situation negative when you do not take control of the thoughts that enter your mind. Make an intentional decision for your mind to work for you and train yourself to only see the positive in any situation. If you adopt this way of thinking into your everyday life, you will automatically see things differently.

We need to focus more on the triggers that cause us to act out. Insecurities are like weeds, they will grow and dominate any area that is not protected and can only be killed by destroying the root. For us to regain our power and rebuild self-esteem, we need to identify where the insecurity stems from and stomp out the root. Like a wild flower, we need pruning to fully bloom without the limiting fears holding us back.

Tips Not to Forget!!!

The passing of the year brings a change to the weather in the form of seasons. The same applies to our life. There is a necessary season for everything and that is something we have to learn to accept and understand. During a rain storm we know it will not last forever. Eventually, the sun will break through the clouds but not until the storm has finished its part. The rain was needed to serve its purpose for the environment and storms in our life are needed to play their part in our journey. We learn and grow from our experiences, good and bad.

Overthinking causes us to create scenarios that are not fact and make things worse by causing self-inflicted anxiety. Taking a moment to settle your thoughts with the facts is beneficial in a pressing situation. When you take your time, you have more control and have the power to ensure a positive outcome.

The final nail in the coffin to kick-start your mind transformation journey is to stop the irrational behaviour that aides life storms. Emotionally fuelled responses only make things worse. Before you respond to that annoying text, put your phone down and distract yourself. I was given the best advice when responding to text messages that test your inner Gandhi. Type out your response but do not press send. Wait at least an hour and nine times out of ten you will end up erasing the message and responding calmly. Try it and see if it works for you!

Most importantly, always remember time is so important especially if it means you can diffuse a situation that will potentially cause permanent damage.

And of course bearing all this in mind, we must not forget the importance that the law of cause and effect has on our lives.

Part Two

The Law of Cause and Effect
–What Does This Even Mean?

**"Every effect has a specific and predictable cause.
Every cause or action has a specific and predictable
effect."**

Basically this means that everything in life is a direct result of a specific cause. You may be thinking how? There are people starving in the world, they did not cause their starvation. How does that even make sense?

The causes in life relate to the decisions made by either ourselves or someone with remote influence over our lives. For example, a world leader decided to go to war which has resulted in mass death, famine and towns and cities ruined. If they had not gone to war, the country may have remained the same but there is always something happening in the background that we are not privy to. Or what about global warming? How we live our lives has resulted in mass increased levels of pollution that has aided to a gradual increase in the Earth's overall temperature. This has led to rising sea levels resulting in more floods, glaciers melting and extreme weather events. The decision can be the tiniest or the largest but the same rule applies. The impact can be significant or subtle but there is still an effect from the cause.

"Every action has a reaction." I learnt this initially when writing scripts. You can never have a character that undertakes an action without an actuality manifesting from that action. Nothing in life or fiction just happens without something else coming from it. Look at the classic Walt Disney film Snow White. The princess had to eat the apple to be poisoned to fall into the deepest sleep which then led to her finding her true love. The cause was the apple and the effect was the protagonist establishing the identity of her true love. Yes, I know that is just a film but this also happens in real life. Ultimately, our decisions lead us to our reality.

Planting analogies are another perfect example to focus on when relating to the relevance that the law of cause and effect has on your life. Soil has no real purpose or benefit until you plant a seed and nurture that seed which later flourishes into something of use.

The product produced from the soil and the quality, all depends on the seed you have planted as well as your efforts in maintaining the growth process. The same applies to your life.

The cause is the thought which acts as the seed planted into our mind which is the soil. If you plant rotten seeds, (thoughts) you will reap negativity (effects) and vice versa. On the contrary, if your effects (reality) are filled with confusion and ambiguity it's a clear sign that you are not filling your mind with progressive thoughts (causes).

If you plant a lemon seed, you will produce a lemon tree that will bear fruit. If you plant apple seeds, then you will benefit from an apple tree. To get the best out of life you need to ensure your planting skills are at their utmost high.

How you live your life right now is the result of the thoughts you have planted that have led to your actions and inevitably your current experiences. Our thought manifestations are vital to the outcome of our lives so we need to ensure the right seeds are being planted on a daily basis.

You can also plant seeds into other people via your actions which will alter how they see you. This is why your mindset is super important! Your leading energy – positive or negative will be a direct result of the type of seeds you have planted within yourself.

This concept relates to different religious ideologies. Firstly, we can look at 'karma'. In its simplest definition, karma is related to the actions people perform and their sentiment behind these actions. We also know it as, "**What**

goes around comes around." The dictionary's definition for karma is the following:

> *The sum of a person's actions in this and previous states of existence, viewed as deciding their fate in future existences.*

My definition is that the intentions of your actions good or bad will return to you in the form of a blessing or a curse. I use the word curse lightly here but it basically means a form of negativity on your life. How you treat other people is, so, important as the law of cause and effect means if you are bad to another person, this needs a direct reaction which will result in bad coming back to you. What you put out you get back, so if you give out bad, it's inevitable what you will receive. It also does not mean it will affect you straight away or in the same way. It is result of an action which has the associated kinetic energy that basically means you have negativity added to your list of unavoidable returns.

In Christianity, the bible verse Galatians 6:7 states:

"A man reaps what he sows. For whatsoever a man soweth, that shall he also reap."

This brings us back to the planting analogy and the importance of the seeds that you sow will result in the quality of your harvest.

The laws don't change across the board and the same rules apply. Cause and effect is very real and we need to start paying more attention to what we are manifesting in and out of our lives.

Tips Not to Forget!!!

We can all remember a time in life when we knew we shouldn't do something but did it anyway and then were dealt with the brunt of our disobedience. Everything in life happens for a reason whether good or bad and it's usually after the pain has settled that we understand the lesson that has resulted in a benefit.

Use diligence and good intentions when planting your seeds and never forget the importance of maintenance when trying to achieve the perfect fruit.

Part Three

Work Hard but Smart – The Importance of Modelling

In business and in life, we are advised to model successful people who have achieved similar goals to what we are currently trying to achieve. A common sense approach is to copy the same process which has worked for them and it will work for you. This is sometimes confused with plagiarism and when it does not work, further confusion fuels us to quit.

What we need to understand is that to model a winning strategy means to delve deeper into how something works. We need to fully get into their mind to comprehend how the person makes their decisions and why they act a certain way. Key points to identify in a model and yourself are:

Decision Making

Prioritising definitely tops the list when it comes to daily decision making. You need to be able to ascertain what decisions should take up most of your energy. Decision making should not be mixed up with actions that formulate a routine. You should be putting your energy into decisions that are leading towards something great; leading you towards reaching your goal.

Once you have decided on your decision priorities, you will then need to ensure you tackle these at pivotal times in your day. Utilisation of time is key. Only you will know the best times throughout the day where your mind is least distracted and your clarity levels are highest. Amazon's founder and 2019's World's richest man, Jeff Bezos makes all his decisions before 10am. He also minimises the amount of important decisions, notably stating, **"If I make, like, three good decisions a day, that's enough."** If we are going to take advice from anyone, it would be from Mr Bezos.

Great preparation is also essential when making decisions. Small decisions such as what we wear and eat should become automatic routines. Inspirational leaders do not waste unnecessary energy on decisions that do not have a lasting impact on their lives. Steve Jobs was a billionaire and was famously known for his simple dress code. He was often photographed in jeans and a black turtleneck.

Obama made history as the first African American President. His secret, when it comes to decision making, is, **"You'll see I only wear grey or blue suits. I'm trying to pare down decisions. I don't want to make decisions about what I'm eating or wearing, because I have too many other decisions to make."**

This is a clear indicator that successful people do not do things by chance. They prepare for the littlest action and utilise their time wisely to ensure they focus on what's most important. Remember, we all have the same twenty-four hours. It's what you do with yours in comparison to another that really makes the difference. Next time you find yourself in a conundrum about clothes or food, think about what Obama or Steve Jobs would do and grab the closest item and start your day.

Another important factor that comes into decision making is evaluating your options. What are the pros and cons of the outcome relating to your decision? A set criteria that is said to work for successful entrepreneurs are − how will it benefit? Is the decision in line with core beliefs? What will be the true impact?

Mark Twain suggests, **"Good decisions come from experience, but experience comes from making bad decisions."** You have to reflect on the past decisions you have made and use that experience as a benchmark when making your final decision. Take your time, have clarity of thought so you can ensure you have not missed anything vital that may impact your decision. Remember, this type of energy and focus should only be steered towards progressive life impacting decisions, decisions that will lead to greater opportunity towards a substantial goal and your life vision.

Vision

"If you talk about it, it's a dream. If you envision it, it's possible but if you schedule, it's real."
Tony Robbins

Without vision there are no actions implemented to take you anywhere. Vision is bigger than your goals; vision defines your goals because they all originate from your vision. Vision is the bigger picture. Who do you want to be? What do you want to be known for? What type of legacy do you want to leave behind? The vision you have for your life should be the first thing you have in check before you can set goals to help you reach your vision. A business plan is based on an individual's vision. You have an idea of what you want to achieve and now write down your steps in the form of a plan and forecasts. Do you have a business plan for your life? Have you followed the same process when it comes to your life achievements?

Another popular route that acts as motivation, when attempting to reach your goals, are vision boards.

A vision board is when you create a collage of images based on your dream life. Many feel vision boards are a motivation tool and different techniques work for different people. Personally, I feel there is a strong chance of becoming distracted by these visual desires and not taking the relevant action to achieve what you are supposedly manifesting. I am more hands on and prefer to take the risk, try and learn from my mistakes and continue moving in a direction led by action.

Based on your personality you need to know what best works for you. What helped me identify my life vision were the answer to these two questions:

Who do I want to be? A role model. Someone who motivates and spreads positivity to those most in need.

How can I do this? Through my writing.

Those were the two most important questions I answered that led me to write this book and take my craft more seriously. I had always been blessed with the gift of being a natural motivator and teamed with my passion for writing, I knew they would come hand in hand to help me achieve my vision and goal of ultimate success. Being someone who steers more towards a practical mindset rather than theoretical, I automatically lead with the actions. First think, what can I do to achieve my vision? This will then define your goals. Remember your goals should be the accomplishments you strive towards that lead to you reaching your life vision. If you are yet to define your life vision, answer these two important life-changing questions:

Who Do I Want to Be?
How Can I Do This?

Once you have answered those questions, think about a talent that comes naturally to you. What do you enjoy doing? How can you use this to assist you on your journey to becoming the person you have noted as wanting to become? Everyone has a gift. Whatever you excel in and find easy to do with little or no assistance, home in on this and build your goals/strategy around the talent in a way that will provide what is needed to meet your vision.

Some may disagree with my opinion that your life's vision should have no time limit but I am going to own it. I believe unlike a goal we cannot tie a deadline to life's vision. When a goal has a deadline, it will definitely push you to want to meet what you have set out within the indicated time associated with that goal. This is obviously a benefit but when it comes to your life's vision, the key word here is LIFE! Your vision shouldn't end until your life does. It is continuous and there is no amount of time that can be given to something that has a forever notion attached. I say that to say this, don't feel rushed, your vision is ever evolving which means you should always be progressing no matter how small.

Action Process

Where do I start! Three words. **JUST DO IT**. Nike's famous trademark needs to be drilled into our brains frontal lobe when it comes to living life. In addition, taking accountability for what you want to achieve by telling other people, will lead to them providing you encouragement with constant reminders. If I had a pound for every time I have told someone who had an idea but was stuck in procrastination mode to just try, I would be a multi-millionaire. You have to act on something for it to be real life. You could read all the positive, self-help books in the world but not actually adopt any of the practices into your life and nothing will change. Change needs action.

Action produces routine and routine produces results. Without taking action how can you expect to make progress, on anything? You have to take the first step and simply try. When you take action, you automatically enter the trial and error stage that is needed for all stages in life. How do you know if something is going to work if you have not tried? This also eliminates time-wasting so you can re-strategize your life's plan when it comes to reaching your goals towards meeting and upholding your life's vision. Note the word upholding.

Maintaining anything once you receive it in my opinion is harder than the achieving part. The upkeep needed to maintain what you have achieved, especially when it relates to consistency, can be extremely difficult. We revel in the idea of working towards achieving something, putting blood, sweat and tears into meeting personal deadlines, pushing harder and harder then BOOM we get there, we make a significant change. The temptation to rest a little sets in and then we suddenly realise the process of preserving the current situation is a lot harder. The hype from a new business may have died down, now what? We need to continue making pivotal changes towards upholding our new found state of existence.

This is why usually consistent music artists are always the most successful. A lot of the time it's not down to your talent, it's the steps you take and the work you put in to uphold your position. We can all think of a one-hit wonder, don't let that be you with your life.

This is why routine is super important. Once you build productive action steps into your routine, you will always commit to these as they become daily habits. A productive action step is a task that you perform that will push you closer to meeting a goal that leads to your vision. Basically, you break your goals down into smaller, attainable tasks. For instance, I knew that to complete this book I had to ensure I committed a minimum of an hour's writing time a day. I also had to ensure I wouldn't miss the gym and didn't want to eat after seven o'clock so I had to change my entire routine to ensure I met my goals. I first had to ascertain what tasks I could not change. Those for me were my office working hours, as I still work a full-time job. I had to fit everything around my working day so instead of focusing on the tasks I couldn't control, I took responsibility over what I could.

I looked at my sleeping pattern. I am not an advocate for a sleep-less-work-harder life. How are you expected to work effectively and efficiently if you are always tired? I know I work well with a minimum of seven hours sleep so I vowed to ensure I would be in bed by ten-thirty latest. Due to having the luxury of being able to drive to work, I knew if I woke up earlier, I could fit in a gym session every day as this would integrate into my daily routine. This also meant my sleeping pattern would not change and I will not miss sleep thus not impacting my productivity. That was my morning sorted. This freed up my evenings which meant when I got home at roughly six o'clock, I could cook my dinner (I only eat fresh meals), eat and be ready to write from seven o'clock. This allowed me to write for up to two hours and then, from nine o'clock, have at least an hour and a half of free time to watch something or read a book. This is taking control of your routine to make it work for you when you are on a journey. There is no time for excuses. In life you make time for what is most important to you and your goals should be a priority.

In my case, I have always been very routine-orientated but if you are the opposite, this maybe what is stopping you from making effective movement in your life. Before building your routine, look at the tasks that cannot be changed and then revolve your daily routine around those. Allow yourself one day in the week where you can just be free, for me that is a Saturday. I literally do whatever I like but the control freak in me does like to plan in advance. I just cannot live my life by chance. Every minute in the day is important even if it is a rest-day.

Finally, I want to remind you that this is the life you have chosen. You have made a conscious decision to better yourself. You made a commitment to achieve greatness, have it be in the field of business or lifestyle; you have decided you want to take control of your destiny. In response to this decision, we need to take responsibility and be accountable for our actions and always remember why we are doing what we are doing when faced with difficult times.

You may not want to wake up in the morning to go to the gym but you know, deep down, the benefit you are receiving. You want to be healthier; you want to release beneficial endorphins that assist your moods.

We are the driving force when it comes to change and with a clear, focused mindset all we need is the assistance of a productive routine that moves us one step closer to reaching our life's vision.

Tips Not to Forget!!!

Success can be predictable if we are aware of what we are doing. If we take the necessary actions and make the right decisions, we will undoubtedly achieve success. Model your approach on a winning method, limit your decision-making and ensure your routine for life has all the productive steps needed to assist your journey of achieving and maintaining your vision for your life.

Part Four

A Disciplined Mind

We all enjoy watching sporting events such as The World Cup, Olympic Games or Wimbledon. Even those who would not usually indulge in sports make an effort to watch some part of the tournaments. We feed our competitive nature whilst watching; we want to see who will win gold, whose country will be most successful. Deep down, we enjoy seeing those who have worked hard towards a goal, winning and the same applies in our lives.

We like to know our hard work, training and sacrifice will account to success and benefit our lives. This is why there is a great level of appreciation to those who contribute to society.

"The harder the conflict, the more glorious the triumph. What we obtain too cheap, we esteem too lightly."

Thomas Paine

To achieve success and reach our goals we need to put in the work. We need to understand that nothing great comes easy and we will always face hardship and battles. The battles we overcome in life shape our character. They ensure we are armed with the right defence mechanisms that come with experience, preparation and discipline.

A disciplined life starts with a disciplined mind. With no discipline, you allow yourself to be susceptible to distracting influences, susceptible to pitfalls that have no space or room on our journey to reaching our goals. Discipline in itself is a discipline and when you do not operate with a disciplined mind, you lose your only control.

"Rule your mind or it will rule you."

Horace

A disciplined mind means if your goal is to save money, firstly you will need to unsubscribe from all those luring sale emails. We all know the ones, the 20%-off-everything-for-one-day-only and you know you should not but something makes you click that link and then before you know it you've spent what you should have saved. We just need to do what we can to minimise the uncontrolled moments and sometimes the best way to do this is to restrict ourselves from the outset.

If you want to lose weight, prepare your meals and do not buy the types of food that will not help you achieve your goal. Have a realistic plan for exercise. If you are not used to working out, do not force yourself to attend the gym five days a week. This is unrealistic and you will, more than likely, quit. However, if you give yourself realistic expectations these will motivate you and when you get into a regular routine, you can increase those days. Nobody is perfect but the key is to train and make progress no matter how small. As long as we see change, we know we are on the right track.

We have to discipline ourselves to make better choices, not detrimental choices but rather decisions that will help us reach our goals and build character. Being decisive is a trait that is empowering and this comes from having a strong mind which comes with practice, training and dedication.

Your daily affirmations form part of your training towards learning how to apply discipline to your thoughts. We are estimated to have approximately 50,000 − 80,000 thoughts a day. 90% of those thoughts are the same ones we had yesterday. This means we have the choice whether we change the cycle of our thought life or remain the same. If one of your thoughts yesterday was you hate your job, today when you get into the office, you will have that same feeling. This will then affect your mood, how you approach and treat others and just your overall energy.

The turbulence in our lives and our reactions to difficult situations always return back to the nature of our thoughts.

The importance of learning how to reverse unhelpful thoughts is imperative on your journey to establishing a positive mindset. Negative thoughts are like a computer virus. Once you open an email or software program the virus will quickly work to destroy everything that crosses its path. The same applies with negativity but the difference is we have more control. We can decide what we do with the thought that comes into our heads. Whether we allow it to take root or if we decide to replace the thought with something that will serve us better. You would not open an email subjected virus so why do we entertain the viruses of our mind.

Human nature is instinctually designed to win and programmed to lose. We have ideas that can work for us but choose to do nothing with these. The thoughts that serve us, we need more of a push to utilise, but can easily implant the thoughts set out to destroy. We choose how to interpret our thoughts and we choose how to behave in accordance with how we think. Our thinking directly affects our emotional state which is why we have to ensure our minds are right to keep our emotions in check and us in control. Being disciplined means taking control of your thought life and holding all accountability for your choices and actions.

When writing this chapter and discussing the relationship with thoughts to your behaviours based on past experiences, I wanted to address the idea of traumas and how you decide if they affect you in a positive or negative way.

We have discussed fear in some detail in an earlier chapter but I wanted to bring it back to light because it's extremely important. Nothing that has happened in your life that has caused you pain due to another person's negative actions is your fault. Hurt people, hurt people and it is unfortunate that you have experienced such wrongdoing. However, it is your fault if you use the event as an excuse not to live your life to the fullest.

I look at someone like Joyce Meyer who was sexually abused as a child by her Father. Joyce lived a turbulent life but decided she would not let her past be a distraction to creating a beautiful future. She allowed her pain and trauma to act as a motivation rather than a limitation. She regained the power over her life and even cared for her Father in his elderly years. Imagine how hard it would have been for Joyce to do all of this but with a determined and disciplined thought life you can overcome anything.

You are entitled to feel like a victim because you are one. Just do not allow a victim's mindset to rob your joy and true potential. The trauma has stolen progressive aspects of your past; do not allow it access to the greatness aligned with your future.

Successful Athlete's Mentality

We need to learn how to adopt a successful athlete's mentality in our everyday lives. Successful athletes concentrate on an upcoming performance and block out any harmful thoughts that forces them to lose focus. They focus on the goal and not on their competitors or any uncontrollable factors.

They move intentionally and throw all their focus on what they can control such as their fitness and state of mind. They focus on being productive. Everything they do, no matter how small, is preparing them to face their next challenger.

They understand the importance of making the right decisions and taking the necessary steps that will aid them in reaching their personal goals. They master the art of persistence and acknowledge their responsibility with committing to this choice of becoming an athlete and everything that the role comes with.

The key to this powerful mindset is practice, implementing thoughts, beliefs and attitudes that aid to greatness rather than defeat, attitudes that build your mental strength and in turn reflect in dedicated persevering action.

Athletes have many strategies that aid them in reaching their goals. I've selected these three strategies used by successful athletes that should be routed in our everyday lives:

1. Practice and Develop Specific Preparation Routines

When you consistently perform a task diligently, eventually you get better at that task. This, combined with preparation and a structured routine, will aid to you achieving great things.

The reality you perceive becomes the end product of your mindset. It is unrealistic to think everyone can be positive all the time but the secret is practicing how to see the good out of bad situations. For example, you maybe grieving due to the loss of a loved one who had a terminal illness. Our initial thoughts and feelings are clouded by the pain felt from the loss. We enter deep sadness and forget about all the good times we shared and the memories that were filled with love.

Yes, grieve and take as much time you need to do so but don't allow the grief to consume you. Redirect your grief towards something that will serve a purpose. The only positive that can be drawn from a scenario this painful is the fact the person is no longer suffering. They are now at peace and have left you with amazing memories. Use those memories and that thought as your comfort and the torchlight needed to guide you down the murky path of death's darkest tunnel.

2. Quick Recovery Following an Unexpected Mistake or Setback

Everyone loses motivation, gets distracted and has lazy moments. The difference is if you continue in your procrastination or if you break the cycle and get back into motion. An athlete will train for months, sometimes years for an event. If they are unlucky enough not to win the competition, they will continue training for the next event and will not give up. We need the same attitude in life.

We cannot control what happens around us but we can control our strength and how we take part. Our strength is built in our minds. We need to tell ourselves to get up when we feel like staying in bed, depressed. We need to put the junk food down when we are trying to lose weight. Of course, allow yourself a treat once in a while and everything in moderation but if you have a goal to drop the pounds–constant burgers and chips from your favourite fast food franchise is not helping.

We need to encourage and motivate ourselves and not rely on others to do so. Low self-esteems are extremely damaging and we need to learn how to love ourselves with no exceptions. Remember, self-motivation is a difficult, but satisfying, quality. When you learn to fully believe in yourself and your abilities, you can persevere through any hardship that comes with life.

3. Seeking Coaching and Learning from Others

Athlete's recognise and communicate emotional issues that maybe a factor in them reaching their peak performance. They have a team of professionals that support and mentor them.

Pride is a limiting trait that needs to be stripped back in order to reach your ultimate life's vision and all weaknesses addressed to become all-round stronger. There is a perceived weakness associated with asking for help. We need to drop all prideful attitudes and accept that by asking for help we are actually seeking to become a better person and this should be seen as a strength rather than a weakness. Turning to someone for help shows you want to move forward and have realised that you need assistance in a particular area to promote self-growth. Nobody can do everything alone. Successful business owners understand that they need to employ those who are top of their fields to perform tasks they cannot. You need people in life to reach certain peaks and they need you.

We need to learn to communicate deep routed personal issues. Working on the hardest parts of ourselves maybe the difference with conquering our mindsets and falling back into a self-commiserative state.

Tips Not to Forget!!!

Without discipline you are not installing control and focus towards achieving an intended goal. If you are not disciplined, you have no rules that form a structure for your behaviour towards a task. We need to be like athletes and use defeat as motivation to go harder! Address your past traumas and use these as an inspiration to produce a better future.

Part Five

Rediscovering Your Identity –Without Social Media

Please, I repeat, PLEASE do not base your real life off of the fabrication that is social media. The definition for social media:

"Website and applications that enable users to create and share content or to participate in social networking."

You can create absolutely anything online. You can depict a life that is not your own and then actually build a persona based on lies that can make you 'Insta' famous. I could spend my day going into different designer stores, making videos, trying on various shoes, and caption 'can't decide'. I can buy something totally different and caption 'had to buy both'. None would be wiser. You then upload your pictures and videos with all the hashtags in the world to ensure you are noticed and just like that you become an influencer.

Social Media is the fastest cause of depression and fake lifestyles are the most counterproductive entity ever to be birthed. There is a proven causal link between the use of social media and having a negative impact on our mental health. There has been a rise in cosmetic surgery spewed from a vanity complex that is associated with a fake image #perfection. On Apps like Instagram, the majority of images you will see are all perfect–filtered personas of the perfect couple, the perfect selfie, a perfect scenery and picture. No one online wants to portray an imperfect life when in reality, life is not meant to be perfect.

Dependent on usage, we make hundreds of comparisons a day to what is seen as perfection and this has a detrimental effect on our mental health. Now, this is in no way intended to be an attack, nor I am trying to sound all high and mighty because, believe me, I love a filter. I just want to push the point that we need to remember not to get obsessed over something that is not a real portrayal of life.

The importance of having your mental health intact is the most underrepresented wellbeing requirement in society today. It is an important aspect for every stage of our life. It is our emotional, psychological and social well-being. It is how we think, feel and act. It leads our choices, reactions and thought processes, in other words it is the microchip implanted in our mindset that needs to function correctly for the remaining processes to all link together to be at their most efficient. It allows us to understand our full potential, cope with life stresses and work productively. It is the first thing to suffer when our defences are at an all-time low and the hardest thing to rebuild once a persistent trigger attempts constant attacks.

We can limit the threats aimed at our mental health by ensuring balance and moderation to anything that acts as a negative influence. We must not be ignorant to the devices that are being used to try and defeat us. If we do not know who we are as individuals, we can easily be swayed by other people's notions and our life's purpose to procreate will be stolen by the negativity associated with a low self-esteem.

For example, when you support a football team, you wear their kit with pride. You sing the songs that are associated with that team; you belong to a culture and follow the behaviours that form the identity of your club. Many of us have lost our identities and no longer know the team we are supporting. We have forgotten who we are and got lost in the ideologies of who we think the internet wants us to be.

Rediscovering our identity needs to include a social media break, especially if we find ourselves becoming distracted by the Instagram likes that mean absolutely nothing in real life but everything online. It is unfair for the younger generation who are growing up with dysfunctional mindsets. What they are being exposed to online, aids to a growing cause of confusion regarding their own manifested identity. We need to be mindful regarding our input online and not get lost in the 'sauce'.

Social Media of course is not all bad. Used in the right way, it can grow businesses, spread positivity and is an effective communication tool for family and friends living in different parts of the world.

"The best way to find yourself is to lose yourself in the service of others."

Mahatma Gandhi

With the struggles of life and the constant need to stay afloat, it is not surprising when we lose our true selves on the journey. Don't allow this to stop you from getting back to your happy place. It happens to everyone and the only game-changing factor is whether or not we manage to get back to our original states by rediscovering our identity. This is a massive benefit when it comes to self-growth and future progression.

To be the best version of you is to really know who you are. How can you be great if you don't know your triggers? You don't actually know why certain actions cause you to behave in a negative destructive way. We need to differentiate from destructive interpersonal, familial and societal influences that do not serve us. Negativity is like a tumour; it produces a domino effect and spreads with its aim to destroy only getting progressively worse without the needed immediate attention.

As mentioned in the chapter regarding your learned fears, you need to enter the realm of discomfort and address the unresolved past traumas that are playing havoc with your future. We must learn to break harmful thought processes, separate negative personality and reject unhelpful defence mechanisms learnt from childhood.

Your identity is not measured by achievements as we already hold great value. It is based on your morals, ideals and beliefs. What means more to you and why? Seeking meaning to life gives us a purpose and this sense of purpose will act as our motivation if and when our crown slips. We all live by different values which is why no two people have the same life. Your core values are the blueprint for your life. They are the structure in place that shapes your integrity and common behaviours.

For instance, if one of your core values is to always treat people with respect, you will have a leading trait of being able to compromise as this is a common association. Look at your leading personal traits, they will assist when establishing your core values and remember there is always room for improvement. We can always adjust our values and make changes where necessary to ensure constant growth.

Ultimately, our goal in life is to be happy. You can have all the money in the world but if you are not happy, what is the point? We see it every day, people with millions of pounds living with a hidden sadness that, unfortunately, consumes them and, sadly, ends in suicide. The moral codes we live by must assist our needs and desires for true happiness. Think about your life, are the core values that you live by aiding to your happiness? If the answer is no, then you may need to readdress these to get you back to that happy place with the aid of professional assistance dependent on your position.

I wrote this book as an aid to open our eyes to unknown limitations that may be holding us back from reaching our true potential. Each of the chapters are intended to unravel uncomfortable truths. In order to move forward we need to address past demons that act as major setbacks. Once we reach this state and we are fully in tune with our strengths and weaknesses. This will open us up to lasting change and prepare us for the final piece of encouragement needed that comes in the form of daily affirmations.

Tips Not to Forget!!!

Social media cannot be the basis of what we deem actual reality. The importance of ensuring you are mentally healthy is paramount in surviving the stresses of life. Seek help where needed and readdress your core values to enable a progressive alignment.

Lastly, we must always remember everything we do in life is to lead us to our ultimate destination which is to be happy and at peace amidst the trials and tribulations of life that will never disappear.

Part Six

Yet vs Now – Now You Are Ready

You are one step closer to making a lasting change to your thought life. We only have one life and we have to make an intentional decision to live this life to the fullest. Our life is based on choices and the importance of making the right choice no matter how difficult. Usually the right choice means applying a level of restraint which can be extremely uncomfortable when we are used to living a certain way.

Yes to YOLO (you only live once) attitude but use this movement to empower not destruct your future. Install the discipline you need to make the right decisions that benefit your life. Never forget, discipline does not bring immediate joy but rather a long-lasting satisfaction.

Positive thinking will not get you to where you want on its own. The formation of your mindset plays a massive part to whether you are going to put into practice what we have discussed. Your patterns in life can only change when your beliefs do. Our beliefs are created from birth to roughly six years old and our lives are a by-product of these beliefs. During this time we also form a mindset based on growth or fixed ideologies.

Carol S. Dweck's (PhD) explanation on mindsets is the most profound and accurate definition I came across when studying for this book. I measured her concept against the areas of my life where my mindset was fixed, and the correlation with stagnant growth and self-inflicted limitation was astounding.

Carol explains the two mindsets like this – Fixed mindset, intelligence is static. It leads to a desire to look smart and therefore a tendency to avoid challenges, easily give up on obstacles, view effort as a waste of time, ignore useful negative feedback and feel threatened by the success of others. As a result those with fixed mindsets may plateau early and achieve less than their full potential. All this confirms a deterministic view of the world.

I used to display a fixed mindset when it came to my stubborn personality trait. I would often use this as an excuse when I did not want to compromise or behave in a way that was progressive towards myself and others. People would know me to be stubborn and would just leave me to it. We also see this when people say things like, "I am stuck in my ways." They have already decided and implied they are not willing to change. We must accept them for who they are and get on with it. When reading, if you stumble upon a word that you don't understand, do you stop and look up the meaning or do you continue reading hoping to make sense of the content without fully teaching yourself something new? These examples plus many more, that I am sure have come to mind, will indicate if you are operating with a fixed mindset in areas of your life.

We then look at the opposing mindset that is based on detecting faults, and generating a process to correct those faults to produce greater results, a growth mindset. Carol describes a growth mindset as − Growth mindset, intelligence can be developed. It leads to a desire to learn and therefore a tendency to embrace challenges, persist in the face of setbacks, see effort as the path to mastery, learn from criticism, and find lesson and inspiration from the success of others. As a result, they reach ever higher levels of achievement. All this gives them a greater sense of free will.

When you lead with a growth mindset, you are constantly on a journey to better yourself. You want to learn because you understand you do not know everything. You do not see a lack of knowledge as a negative in your life or allow this to impact your self-esteem. Failure is not seen as an evidence of unintelligence but rather used as motivation to succeed. Out of the two mindsets which one are you leading with?

Both of these mindsets created from a young age formulate our behaviours and relationships with failure and success in both professions and personal contexts. They also define our capacity for accepting the levels of contentment associated with our happiness.

How a child is praised holds immense dictation on which mindset they create. Studies show children who are praised directly for their intelligence rather than their process tend to grow with a fixed mindset, and those praised for their process and efforts grow with growth mindsets. As parents and guardians, bear this in mind the next time you congratulate your child on their homework.

Now that this has been highlighted, don't panic as it is never too late to change your mindset. Your brain can be developed like a muscle. The harder you train a muscle the more it will grow and become defined. The same applies to the knowledge implanted in your brain. For your brain to get stronger it relies on what you feed it. Read more, become process driven towards challenges and your mindset will change to allow you to be more free-willed in thinking. Transform the meanings of effort and difficulty in your mind, and make obstacles work as an opportunity for growth rather than a restriction.

Now you have an idea of the importance and what you need to do to get your mind right, let us talk about the power of words and how what you say to yourself can make or break you.

The information fed to our subconscious mind is what it uses to operate. If you tell yourself it is difficult to get money, your subconscious will present illusions of obstacles that will assist your goal in not making any money. However, if you tell yourself you will make more money this year compared to the amount made last year, your mind will make you see every opportunity as having the potential of being extremely lucrative. You need to allow your words to serve you daily and stop planning problems with what we say.

Using empowering words like 'I will' act as a conviction to actions you want to perform. Steering away from nonconcrete words such as 'I should, I wish, I hope' in relation to making a change in your life will assist with formulating a new blueprint for your mind to follow. Your mind will do its job when you instruct it to. We are told to be specific with our requests to get the most out of an expectation. If you are redecorating your house and a painter asks you what colour you want to paint your walls and you say, "Any colour, you choose." To your surprise, you come home to lime green walls but was hoping they would be magnolia. How can you be angry at the painter when you did not give clear instructions? The same applies to your mind. You need to give clear instructions for what you want your mind to do and it will follow through.

This is why we need to take full accountability for the words we feed our subconscious. When you speak out a negative, your mind will create further negatives. If someone asks about your day at work and every day you reply 'draining', eventually you will notice you start to feel rundown. Your body is doing what you are telling it to do.

Challenge yourself, try something different and see how it works for you. Find all the negative words you use regularly and switch it around and use the positive version. Try and change all the negative words you are using concerning yourself, and use the opposing term and see if it changes your overall approach to life and your actions. Instead of saying you are forcing yourself to finish a book, say something like I am really enjoying reading this book; I am looking forward to seeing what happens at the end. Automatically, your association to the task has changed and it has gone from being a chore to finish to exciting. Your body and efforts will react to the task differently.

The mind believes what we tell it. It will respond to the pictures and words we have installed so it is up to us to ensure we create empowering images for the mind to revert back to. If you constantly say things like, "I am so fat. My weight is the reason why I do not have a boyfriend," your mind will allow you to believe this and when men do approach you, you will automatically have this thought leading your actions and behaviours. This is counterproductive on your self-esteem and in your search for love.

Self-praise needs to be our biggest familiarisation. Praise from other people assists and sometimes solidifies our views on ourselves, but these can be masked with selfish agendas for their gain from our insecurities. We need to learn to stop criticising ourselves and boost our self-esteem by praising the things we love about ourselves. The simplest things we must learn to praise, good and bad. Yes, I might have some extra flab on my stomach but that does not take away the fact I am a strong, beautiful woman. There are so many things that we feel insecure about that we need to reprogram our mind on its views. If you cannot think of any good traits about yourself, start with knowing and believing you are ENOUGH. God made you with unique qualities that only you have. Only you sneeze the way you do. You are the only person in this world with your smile, walk and mannerisms that in itself makes you very special.

Familiarisations are important for our self-development because they act as our safety net. We all remember, as a child, wanting a particular item that gave us comfort. We also see regularly, parents using pacifying techniques when a child has a temper tantrum, putting on a favourite film or song and instantly the child quietens. This is all part of a familiarisation we have formed to link us with our mind pleasures.

If your current familiarisations are not working to help advance your character, you can change the picture associations and make only positives familiar and negatives unfamiliar. Remember you always fall back on what is familiar to you.

A good example of the affects this has on your mind is your associations to pain with the familiar triggers you have created. If you have told yourself, "You will never find a good partner," when you meet someone who displays the noted qualities, like someone who shows you love, is loyal and communicates well, you will automatically reject this. Common words that follow self-rejection in this area are 'he/she is too good for me'. The reason why we cannot accept something good is simply due to the idea that we are not used to it. We are not familiar with this kind of behaviour from the opposite sex and usually end up messing up the relationship and running back to the dysfunction we are familiar with.

Your mind feels most comfortable around familiarisations where we have created a safe association. A safe association does not always mean safe as in no immediate physical danger but it means safe to us. What we fall back on and what we need to make us feel comfortable in an uncomfortable situation.

This is why daily affirmations aid in assisting our minds to reconfigure the associations and pictures painted. In times of stress, our imaginations defeat all forms of logical thinking. You can do the same thing every day but a change in circumstance can change everything.

In cases where you have to speak publicly or act on a stage, you could have practiced profusely and have all the experience but as soon as it's show day and you walk on the stage, the intensity from the spotlight beaming on you, your imagination starts playing tricks, thoughts start to enter your mind like, "What if the audience laughs at me? What if I forget my lines?" and just like that you have stage fright and cannot remember any of your words. Subconsciously, you told your thoughts to work against you. You told yourself the audience would laugh at you and you had forgotten your lines, so your body made sure it followed your instructions.

If you had a series of strong, empowering words engrained in your psyche from your daily affirmations, they would act as a safety net. If your thoughts had fell onto words like, "I am strong, I can overcome any obstacle," this would aid your confidence and ultimately paint a different picture for the reality that was cascading due to uncontrolled nerves.

I see affirmations as positive beliefs that are repeated to remind you how great you are! That is not the dictionary definition but that is my definition! They are words we use to remind ourselves of our strengths and serve as a constant reminder of our baptised identity.

To affirm something is to believe in its truth. You have faith and confidence in what you are saying and in turn you are forming your subconscious mind on positive connotations based on how you see your life. If you form your subconscious with positive affirmations, eventually your mind will align those thoughts with your reality hence the reprogramming element associated with daily affirmations.

As with every intentional action you need to first prepare and we have reached the end of the preparation period. If you have followed all the tips highlighted in this book, you should already feel enlightened and excited to make the change needed to make a difference in your life. One of the purposes of this book is to aid with the reprogramming of your mind, and erase all current negative glitches to ensure you only see the positive in even the worse of situations.

I wanted to write something that would be the perfect **'go to'** for an added boost of motivation needed to get through life's struggles. With everything happening in the world today, often we do not take the necessary time needed to really address our own needs. There are so many of us suffering in silence and lacking in the self-support that can get us through any trial.

Always remember, the mind is our most powerful asset and keeping this in check will aid to our confidence in self-love and happiness.

The next stage of the book features daily affirmations with short breakdowns. It is definitely worth writing personal affirmations that focus on the areas in your life that you most struggle with. The next thirty pages will have affirmations for thirty days to kick-start your journey.

Read one affirmation a day, out loud, and repeat the words throughout the day when you have weak moments.

Keep this book in your bag, in your drawer at work, anywhere you can easily get to it when times feel hard.

I want the words to be an encouragement to you and also act as a helping hand as you start the journey towards learning how to self-motivate.

Take this book everywhere and read it repeatedly until your mind's blueprint has been reconstructed, and leads with the positive energy you deserve and your destiny needs. IT CAN HAPPEN AND IT WILL!

DAY 1

The Affirmation — Say it out loud!

It's through adversity that my true character is revealed. I am stronger through my adversity! With every trial I face, I get stronger!

The Breakdown:

Remember what you go through in life moves you one step closer to achieving your goal. We need challenges to fully unravel our true character. I will look at my struggles, hard times and battles as learning processes that teach me new things about myself. I am getting stronger and wiser with each mishap that comes my way and I will not allow the bad times to get me down. I will smile when affliction presents itself and welcome it. I know it has been brought to me as a blessing rather than a curse.

DAY 2

The Affirmation − Say it out loud!

I must remember, in life there is a season for everything. No matter what I am experiencing it will pass and things will get better! Nothing bad lasts forever.

The Breakdown:

Everything in life has a reason and a season. Seasons mean change and change is needed to bring progress. My thoughts need to be aligned with greatness so no matter what I am going through I know there is light at the end of the tunnel. Adverse seasons will bestow onto me greater appreciation for favourable seasons. With all things I must be grateful for life, thankful to see another day and remain in this sentiment always and forever.

DAY 3

The Affirmation – Say it out loud!

My mind can either work for me or against me! Today my mind will work for me.

The Breakdown:

My life is a product of my thoughts and my mind is my strongest fighting force. I generate my thoughts with my environment playing a massive influence in my thought life. I must learn to block out any thoughts that have a limiting or defeating purpose. I have been born into this world to make a positive difference and my thoughts need to align with my actions. Anything that happens in my life today and in the future, I will only see the blessing in that situation. I will only focus on the beneficial aspects and will use these to help push me closer to achieving my goals.

DAY 4

The Affirmation − Say it out loud!

When I think positively, I can see the potential in every situation. There is always a lesson to learn!

The Breakdown:

I must remember a situation has the potential of going two ways. Good or bad. I have the power to make sure it only goes positively. I must use my past experiences as lessons to help me in life when I face a similar crisis. Tough times produce the best results and are the greatest teachers! Next time I am faced with a difficulty I will enjoy the process it takes for me to overcome the trial.

DAY 5

The Affirmation − Say it out loud!

Positive thinking gives me power over any circumstance!

The Breakdown:

Instead of pandering to any uncomfortable moments, I must confidently confront the problem head on and remember no matter the circumstance, I will always win because I set the standards. I make the rules when it comes to my life and how I choose to live it. If I steer through life with a winning mindset, I will always come out of any circumstance, triumphant.

DAY 6

The Affirmation – Say it out loud!

In a crisis, I must always keep my mind focused and not allow my mind to wander.

The Breakdown:

I must look at all aspects of an argument or a heated discussion. I must learn to understand that different people think and act differently to how I think and act. We are all unique individuals and react to things in our own special way. I must take time to act in situations that cause me to feel emotional or uncomfortable. If I give it time, I can diffuse something that could have potentially caused permanent damage.

DAY 7

I must filter out the bad thoughts and only allow in good thoughts. It all starts with what I think!

The Breakdown:

My life is the result of my thoughts becoming actions. Before my feet hit the ground and I start walking, the thought automatically goes into my mind that I need to get up and walk. I must remember I do not do anything in life without it first starting as a mere idea. Good thoughts are based on good experiences and these need to take the lead in my thought life. When a negative thought is trying to creep in, I need to push in the good thought before the bad even has time to settle and grow.

DAY 8

In the same way I take responsibility for my actions, I must take responsibility of my thoughts!

The Breakdown:

I am responsible for what I think and from today I promise to take full control. If I decide to think negatively, I have allowed this and I must accept that responsibility. If I want change, I must first initiate it. We are all given the same level of control over our lives but it's how we implement the control that makes the difference. It's all birthed in the mind and will manifest into greatness or nothingness. I choose GREATNESS!

DAY 9

Filling my mind with the good life has to offer, blocks out the bad!

The Breakdown:

If I strengthen my mind with good memories, they will act as a weapon when I have weak negative moments. Good always overcomes bad so be armed with happy thoughts and they will paint new pictures in your mind when bad thoughts try to creep in. I must not and will not allow fake, negative notions steal my joy.

DAY 10

I control my emotions!

The Breakdown:

Think about something that makes you smile. Now smile. It is as easy as that. Our minds are powered by thoughts that can change any emotion. I can change how I am feeling even if the emotion is not aiding to progress. I need to stop giving outside influences the control and snatch my power back. My emotions will not rule me! I rule them.

DAY 11

The Affirmation − Say it out loud!

My mind is built on positive foundations!

The Breakdown:

My mind needs to be formed from the strongest of foundations. Just like any building, the structure is only as strong as the foundations that keep it in place. If my mind is formed on positivity and goodness, it will mean when I stumble and my thoughts begin to steer towards negativity, I will always have an uplifting safety net of victory rather than destruction.

DAY 12

The Affirmation − Say it out loud!

Today is a new day. Today is a good day! I can and will achieve all that is set out for me.

The Breakdown:

I have the power to ensure my day goes the way I want it to go. I have the power to achieve every goal I set out to achieve. I must remember to be diligent and intentional with every action, emotion and encounter that comes my way. If I start my day knowing it will be a good day, then it will be a good day. This is a choice we are given and I choose to run with it and make every action count and work to my benefit.

DAY 13

My mind is focused and my heart is ready to accept good things and happiness!

The Breakdown:

Gone are the days I will allow myself to feel as though I do not deserve good things and happiness. No matter my circumstance or my past, I deserve to be happy and to be loved. I will open my heart to new opportunities that will lead to long-lasting joy and fulfilment.

DAY 14

The Affirmation − Say it out loud!

I am a winner and can achieve my goals with a focused mindset.

The Breakdown:

I will remember that when it comes to achieving my goals, it's all about the planning and the process. It's the small steps that lead to the big improvements. Over time, with a focused and deliberate mindset, I will develop a strategy that will lead me to always win. I will stay true to my vision and procreate winning models with my own flare and adapt on these where necessary.

DAY 15

My challenges will not defeat me! My challenges will empower me!

The Breakdown:

My past does not dictate my future. I will thrive with new strengths gained from overcoming my challenges. I will respond to each and every challenge with optimism and determination whilst using my past experiences as future aids. Every hurdle I have overcome has led me to this day and my strength attracts ongoing opportunity.

DAY 16

I will persevere. I will not quit.

The Breakdown:

I must always remember that my life means something. I was born for a unique reason. When times feel hard, I have to keep going and use my inner strength as motivation. I must stop allowing circumstances to bring me down and feel as though I am are not good enough. I am more than enough! I believe if I continue to work hard, think positively, and take the right steps, I will achieve my goals. Perseverance makes me stronger and is a clear indication that I can overcome any hurdle that comes my way.

DAY 17

I will stop waiting for something good to happen. I will think goodness into my existence and be assured that good things ARE coming my way!

The Breakdown:

I create the causes that turn into the effects that affect my life. I can think goodness into my life and goodness will be attracted to me. I can choose to see an opportunity in every situation and I will decide to utilise this opportunity. I need to leave the days behind where I would be miserable and simply wait for good times. I must not forget, I create the good times! I am the co-author of my life and play a massive part in controlling how everything plays out.

DAY 18

The Affirmation − Say it out loud!

Today I pledge to only concentrate on the good in my life! I will be decisive about my happiness and will not allow anything negative to change my outlook.

The Breakdown:

I control and dictate my happiness. I decide what I focus on and have complete control over my feelings. There is so much good in my life! I have been blessed with the gift of life and promise to live a life of meaning and appreciation.

DAY 19

The Affirmation – Say it out loud!

Success will be manifested into every aspect of my life

The Breakdown:

I will see every opportunity as a means of success. Every task that I complete leads me towards reaching my life's vision. I am on the road of constant progression and no action is a wasted task.

DAY 20

The Affirmation − Say it out loud!

I am strong enough to overcome any battle that presents itself.

The Breakdown:

"That which does not kill us makes us stronger." − Friedrich Nietzsche. This saying will be implanted in my mind whenever I face challenges that are trying to defeat me. I will always remember that my strength grows with each battle in life that I overcome. The satisfying feeling I will get once I overcome this challenge will serve as my motivation. I will remember that I am given these battles as hurdles needed to pass and they will benefit my character in the long run.

DAY 21

I am in love with myself. It does not concern me how another person feels about my presence.

The Breakdown:

I will not allow other people's negative words about me influence my life. They are entitled to an opinion and I choose to ignore anything that is not intended to bring progress, love or positivity. I am fully in love with every aspect of myself and will maintain this feeling at all times.

DAY 22

The Affirmation – Say it out loud!

I am blessed and highly favoured.

The Breakdown:

I was born to do great things. I am blessed in every aspect of life and will choose to see the blessings daily. God has granted me favour to ensure I will succeed no matter what comes my way. God's promises for my life will come to pass and I will live by faith and hope that tomorrow will provide further blessing and grace.

DAY 23

The Affirmation – Say it out loud!

I will not let my doubts stop me from trying! There is no room for excuses, only results!

The Breakdown:

Diligent action produces results and I will take full responsibility for my actions. I will put in the work necessary to fulfil my life's purpose. Doubts have no place in my mind and hold no power over my mindset and self-judgement.

DAY 24

Rejection has no power over me.

The Breakdown:

Rejection is a normal part of life. I will no longer allow the fear of rejection to act as a deterrence to life's wants. I will receive and accept what is supposed to be for me and serve a purpose in my life. If I do not get what I want, it was not meant for me in the first place and I will move on joyfully.

DAY 25

I will not allow the fear of progression to steal my joy.

The Breakdown:

Fear has no place in my heart or mind. My happiness comes from me knowing I will always win. I will hold no fear in trying to move forward in life. I know I will meet obstacles but they will assist my journey. Fear will not steal my purpose and I will not cooperate with self-destruction by giving unnecessary fears any power.

DAY 26

I am not a victim to my circumstances.

The Breakdown:

My past has helped to get me where I am today. I am grateful for my experiences and will use these as motivations for a better future. I am a fighter and nothing will stop me from reaching my true potential in life. Thank you to my aggressors for being my inspiration to do better.

DAY 27

The Affirmation – Say it out loud!

I am enough.

The Breakdown:

I am comfortable within myself and my identity. I have nothing to prove to anyone and bring value to those in my life. I know who I am as a person and I love every aspect of my being.

DAY 28

I will align my wants with my beliefs

The Breakdown:

Life does not give you what you want; it gives you what you believe. I must align my beliefs and my emotions to ensure they always work for me. I am the only force stopping myself from achieving so I need to regain control.

DAY 29

The Affirmation – Say it out loud!

**I will display empathy and compassion towards
everyone I meet.**

The Breakdown:

I must learn to become more tolerant when interacting
with different types of people. I will embrace other people's
way of life and always show respect and love through my
actions. I will learn to see life from different perspectives and
will enhance my communication by adapting my approach
and making a conscious effort not to judge.

DAY 30

The Affirmation – Say it out loud!

My anxieties will not take hold of my life.

The Breakdown:

From today and for the rest of my life, I will live without worry, anxiety and fear. Today is the beginning of a new me. Worry free! I am the author of my life and can create goodness by not focusing on negatives. I manifested all my anxieties and I cast them out of my life and refuse to be a victim to a fear that does not exist.

**Transformed, Empowered and Ready
To Live Your Best Life!**

Now that you have followed all the steps and performed the daily affirmations you are ready to step into the world with new eyes. I believe in order to live to your fullest you need to be armed with the right mentality to view life from multiple viewpoints.

We need to remain vigilant, in control and in constant pursuit of our happiness. Live intentionally, do not give up when times feel tough, and build your own approach that allows you to deal with the inevitable trials that will arise to test you.

Always think on purpose, discipline your mind and take control of your thoughts. When people say things like, "I am a product of my environment," they are incorrect. We are products of our thoughts and no matter what your circumstance you can change your future by taking control of all areas of your thought life.

I hope you have found solace, encouragement and motivation in this book to challenge yourself, deal with unresolved personal demons, and take the steps you need to mould you a better life. I will leave you with this bible verse from James 1:4, **"Let perseverance finish its work so that**

you may be mature and complete, not lacking anything."
Good luck and enjoy the journey!